Live Life Laughing

An Innovative and Imaginative Approach to Living A Healthier, Happier, and Prosperous Life

By

Rosalind H. Trieber, MS, CHES, NFL
The Naturally Funny Lady

Illustrations by Suzi Moffatt

Cover Design by Yale Bernstein

Published by

Trieber Associates, Inc.

Owings Mills, Maryland

Trieber Associates, Inc.

P.O. Box 601

Owings Mills, Maryland 21117

410-998-9585 · Fax: 410-356-5921 · e-mail:

New Website & E-Mail:
www.humorfusion.com
roz@humorfusion.com

ISBN: 0-9627329-2-3

Published by: Trieber Associates, Inc. P.O. Box 601, Owings Mills, Maryland

Dedication

To Bernie, for his sustaining love and special wisdom, for his understanding of the way I walk this earth, and most of all – for his complete acceptance of life with a naturally funny lady.

WARNING

This book is for people who need a little nudging to bring out their PLAYFUL ATTITUDE. It is possible they may have lost it by the time they reached the second grade. Silliness, laughter and clowning around were not acceptable criteria for successful graduation. As a result, the attitude of seriousness and accuracy prevailed through adulthood.

Use this book to eliminate terminal or professional seriousness and help make your life happier. Look for the "laughter buddie" for specific instructions to see the funny side and seize an opportunity to laugh at life. Side effects include increased laughter at unexpected times, elevated mood, making other people laugh, increased self-respect and increased energy.

Those who have read this book experience silliness and fun daily!

Proceed with Caution!

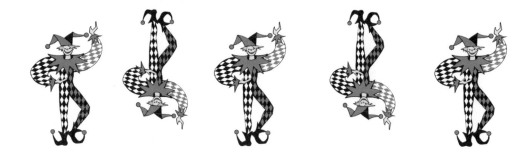

Start Here: What This Book Is All About

Where is it written that Life has to be serious? There is not one single shred of scientific evidence that life is serious. *Live Life Laughing* focuses on your success coming from connecting your mission to your sense of humor. It is 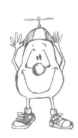 about seeing the funny and absurdity in life instead of the frustrating, adding pleasure to others' lives, avoiding life-o-sucters (people who suck the life out of you, and hanging around with people who make you laugh.

I wrote this book to help you discover how to have fun 365 days a year. *Live Life Laughing* is not a joke book. It is a guide to elevating caring for ourselves and one another to the same kind of art form that we have raised machines and technology. It is about saying, "I don't think so" to life's drainers and embraces the experiences that nurture our creativity and capacity to love.   We seem to place more importance on science and machines than we do our children, our elders and our friends. To think, life is a banquet and half the world is starving!

Humor is serious business. According to C. W. Metcalff, author of *Lighten Up - Survival Skills for People Under Pressure,* humor is a way of being, seeing and interacting with the world. Having a sense of humor gives you the permission to bring out the child within, to be ready for a song, a laugh, a story. Just in case you're having trouble finding your funny bone, I'll help you look for and create humor out of life itself.

Twelve months a year, you can experience the magic of laughter. It doesn't matter if you are watching Eddie Murphy in "The Nutty Professor" for pure enjoyment or a vintage version of "The Three Stooges" as you get chemotherapy; physical and mental health advance to new heights. Your immune system improves, abdominal muscles get an aerobic workout, blood pressure and heart rate are reduced, and circulation improves because of increased oxygen exchange. Blood glucose and cholesterol levels drop to a new low. Who would believe a hearty belly laugh can reduce stress hormones! It happens when you are laughing at the jokes your favorite comedian just told and you can barely help from wetting your pants. And, if you are the moody kind, laughter will help change those razor sharp comments into quick wit in a flash. Laughter is powerful!

Stress destroys and humor heals. **Humor is Empowering.** It takes your mind off of your troubles and eases the pain. It's making lemonade out of lemons. Humor provides us with a new vantage point and helps us detach from the part that wants to be serious. What are you waiting for? Laugh now; avoid the rush!

Were you labeled the "class clown" and told to "wipe that smile off your face and get serious" or did you fail kindergarten because you couldn't color inside the lines? Did you think creativity and thinking were now misdemeanors? Humor comes to the rescue. Thinking and creative ability are improved when placed in a good - humored atmosphere (you remember-vanilla ice cream covered with a thin chocolate coating). That's right. Genuine scientific studies demonstrate that people become more creative working in an environment of high energy and are stimulated by fun and laughter. The Journal of Educational Psychology reported a study, conducted by A. Ziv, who found that adults became more creative following a concert of humorous recordings. Research has also demonstrated that when a task is framed as "play" rather than work, participants become more effective and creative problem solvers.

As I described the following study in *43 Ways To Keep You and Your Taste Buddies Happy – Outrageous and Hilarious Humor Laced In Between 43 Healthy, Delicious Recipes,* a humorous cook book I co-authored, I describe it to you here as well.

Dr. Arthur Van Gundy of the University of Oklahoma, a known authority in the field of creativity, conducted a study with college students comparing the effect of two different types of environment on the ability to come up with ideas for new snacks: chips, pretzels, etc. One group was in an average classroom and told to brainstorm ideas. The other group was in a room with loud music, good food and Nerf™ guns. The fun-stimulated group came up with 310 ideas while the traditional brainstorming group came up with 29 ideas. The results speak for themselves. Give us fun and games and we will generate more energy and productive ideas than the EverReady ™ Battery.

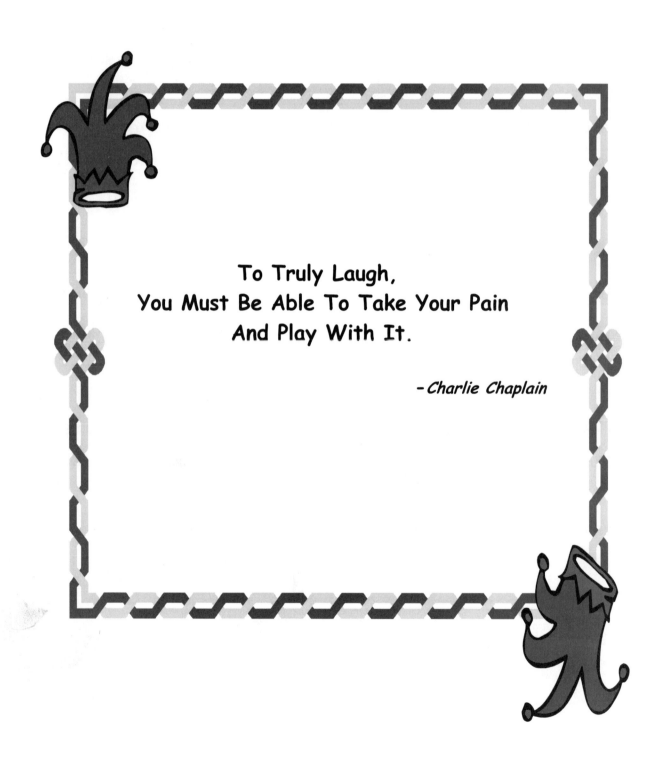

To Truly Laugh,
You Must Be Able To Take Your Pain
And Play With It.

- Charlie Chaplain

Before you reject this idea, engage in a hearty laugh before you pick an argument with your spouse about your mother – in – law moving in or you have to meet with a belligerent client. Natural painkillers, endorphins, are raised and you can stay focused on whatever you are doing. You may decide not to shoot and come up with many other solutions like buying your mother –in - law a one - way ticket to Never - Never Land. You are no longer trapped in a toxic energy dump.

A sense of humor helps us see new possibilities in difficult situations; it reduces the pressure, allowing us to look for an effective solution. Finding the funny side is the vehicle to change the perceptions of our circumstances before they change us. Humor is having the ability to hope for something better or just have fun in the moment. Don't forget, if everything is perfect, there is no comedy. Only when you're all dressed –up at the gala and step out of the restroom with toilet paper stuck to the bottom of your shoes is when there is comedy.

Discover your mission and play with your imagination to find the humor perspective from which to view your stresses. Lighten up under pressure, avoid the hurrying habit, balance work, self and others, and prevent terminal professionalism.

By choosing humor you will live a happier life even when your rented car dies in the middle of the Mohave Desert and it takes three hours to get a replacement car. Just imagine you're on the "Enterprise" and Scotty beams you up out of harm's way!

Smoke Gets In Your Eyes

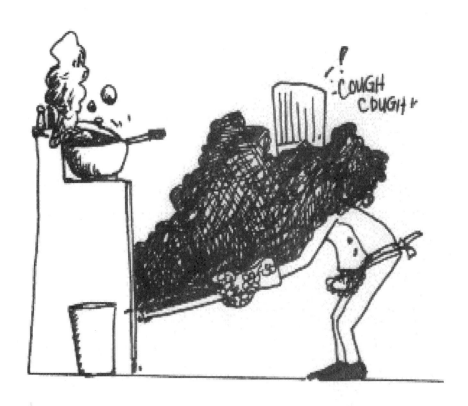

How Long Do You Want To Be Miserable?

The Balance Challenge

You've got twenty-four hours every day to feel like an arrow shot from a cross bow, speeding through an unnoticed present into an unknowable future, afraid of that stone wall target at the end. Or, are you confident about how you want your life to feel at the end of every day that you are able to **balance** between self-care, care for others and work? Can you find the humor in day - to - day experiences?

What does balance have to do with living life laughing? Once you know what your mission is, what you want to be remembered for, you will be able to live life according to your own fun - filled script. The majority of people today live from task to task and paycheck to paycheck. Not exactly a formula for living a successfully productive life embodied with good health, good humor and the feeling of having made a difference.

Maggie Bedrosian, in her book *Life Is More Than Your To – Do List*, suggests you write down the first 10 words that come to mind when asked the question "How Do You Feel When You're Feeling Really Well?" When you feel really well as you described, you function at your optimum. Your creativity and problem solving skills are at their peak. The peak goes even higher when you're in fun. You are not caught up in emotional traps. You are able to handle whatever life hands you with far less stress and anxiety.

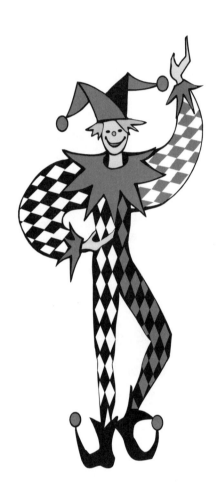

"No Matter How Cynical You Get,

It's Impossible to Keep Up."

-Lily Tomlin

If you suffer from emotional constipation, you might have trouble answering that question. Let me put it to you another way. Visualize yourself going on vacation resentfully taking your laptop computer and joyfully taking your golf clubs. You are feeling over – worked, exhausted and looking forward to a stress free, work free vacation. Unfortunately, unfinished reports need to be completed. This now becomes a "working" vacation. The computer weighs only five pounds, the golf clubs over thirty pounds. Which would you rather be carrying? At this point, you are going on a vacation half - heartedly. Which would you rather be —overworked or underplayed? Get the point?

Having FUN is fundamental to living a meaningful life.

Take a break, stop whenever you find yourself missing the adventurous experiences each day brings. If you feel overwhelmed, stop and smell the chocolate candies sitting on your desk, keep a can of silly putty in your desk drawer, pull it out and play with it. Call your secretary, your lover or your kids and say "thank you." You might even pay the toll for the person behind you on your way home.

"The Hardest Thing To Learn In Life Is Which Bridge To Cross And Which To Burn"

-David Russell

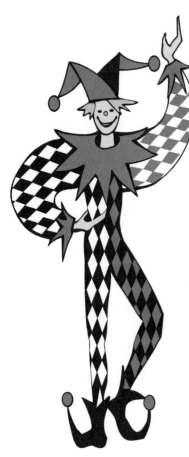

No Matter How Old You Are

May You Never Stop Shopping

In The Toy Store.

WHAT DO YOU NEED FOR BALANCE?

When was the last time you took the time to even consider what makes you feel good? Take this opportunity to identify what energizes you -what makes you who you are.

 Answer the following questions: Use these pages to write on or make copies for yourself, your family or co-workers.

1. What life experiences fill your heart?

2. What supports your positive self-concept?

3. What nurtures your capacity to love?

4. What drives your creativity?

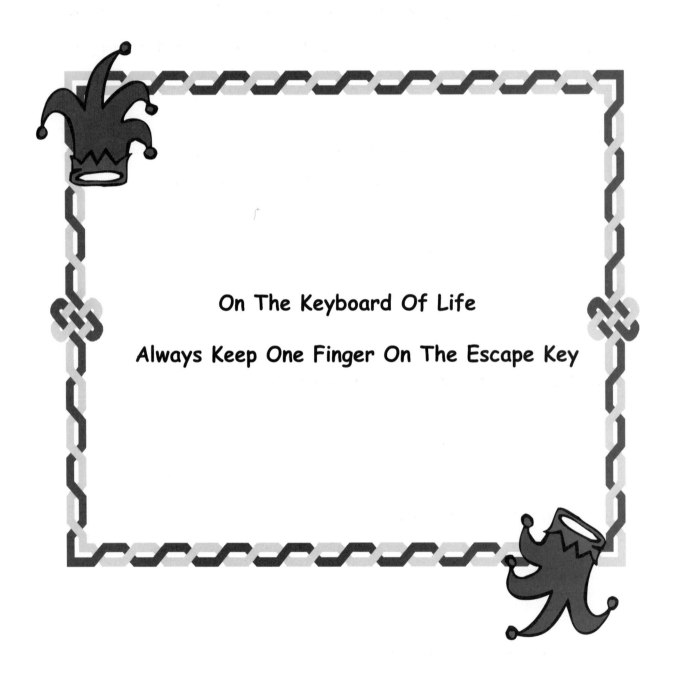

On The Keyboard Of Life

Always Keep One Finger On The Escape Key

5. What motivates your productivity?

6. What people / places / activities invigorate you?

7. When you feel drained, what restores you?

Need some help?

Here are some examples of energizers: watching a sunset, getting a massage, receiving compliments from your spouse or taking a long, leisurely walk. Other fillers could be people, places or activities that bring you joy, stimulate you, give you meaning or make you laugh at home, work or play.

On the other hand, you might want to identify those life – o – sucters, otherwise known as personal drainers.

8. What people, places or activities at home, work or play annoy you, anger you, depress you, wear you out, worry you, frustrate you or

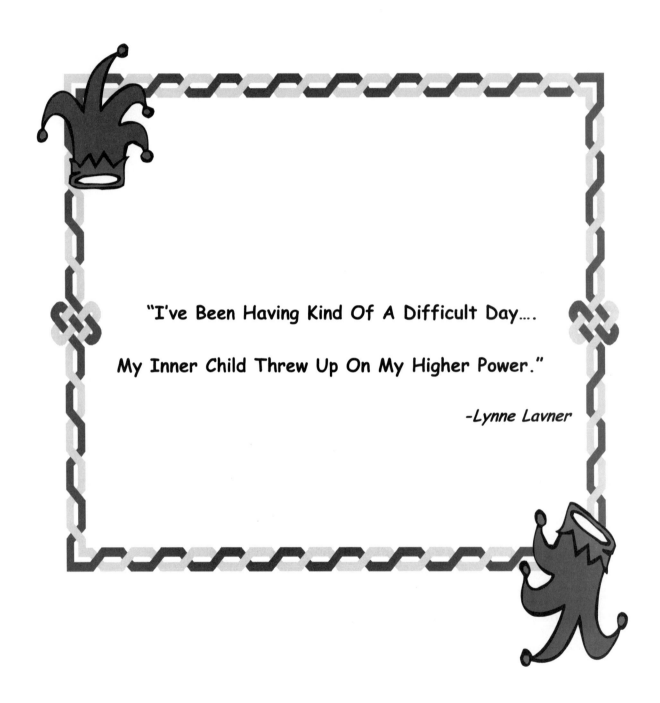

"I've Been Having Kind Of A Difficult Day....

My Inner Child Threw Up On My Higher Power."

-Lynne Lavner

bore you? This could be your whole life! It is possible you may need several pages to answer these questions. Just do it! It all depends on how long you want to hold on to your misery. Once you discover what your life-o-sucters are you need to know how to drain the swamp. After all how many alligators do you want to hang around with?

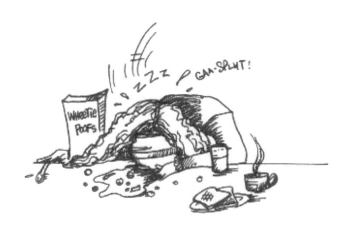

Your Morning Wake-Up Call

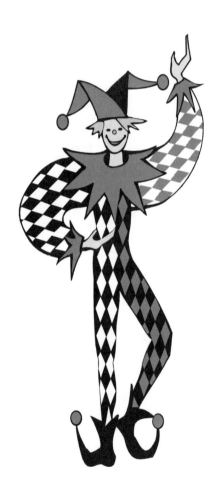

Lost Your Sense of Humor?

Look in the mirror and you will see a message that goes something like this:

*"I don't remember what I wanted to be when I grew up...
But I know it wasn't this."*

If You're Not Having Fun, Doing What Your Doing, Stop Doing It!

TAKE THE BALANCE CHALLENGE

The healthy balance takes different forms. You make a decision about what's important and then you make sure your day – to - day choices implement those decisions (otherwise known as Living Your Mission).

HEALTHY BALANCE GOALS

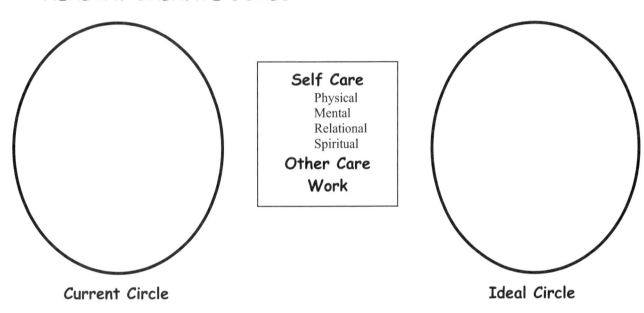

Self Care
Physical
Mental
Relational
Spiritual
Other Care
Work

Current Circle

Ideal Circle

Divide Your Circle

Currently, how would your balance circle look? How do you spend most of your time?

How would you divide your ideal circle?

What would you consider to be the healthiest balance for you? Compare your ideal balance circle to your current balance circle.

What specific observations can you make about your personal preferences and your current balance level?

Why Is There Not One Moment
We Can Call Our Own?

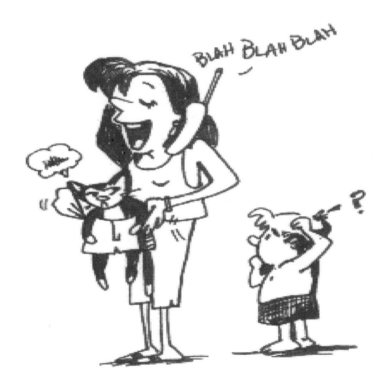

Because the Minutes are Not Hours

I Don't Have An Attitude Problem,

You Have A Perception Problem!

Attitude is everything. Mae West lived into her eighties believing she was twenty, and it never occurred to her that her arithmetic was lousy.

The key to the palace is not under the mat; it is in your attitude! You choose your attitude; attitude is your responsibility. How willing and able are you to invest your time and energy with whole - heartedness to perform one act of kindness, make somebody's day with a smile or a story about the beauty of sharing life's milestones? The only thing that is real is perception. Humor is your unique vision of life, your struggles, your losses and your recovery by discovering and appreciating absurd ideas that allow you to laugh at life.

Humor is attitude. It is a way of thinking, an approach, an outlook and a mindset, even your thoughts. Humor is a form of enjoyment.   Humor researcher Paul McGhee describes humor in the following way: *"We are enjoying an experience that does not fit our mental patterns."* Humor often thrives on the negative condition. It gives you an opportunity to be at odds with the rules of "official society."   Humor helps you laugh at yourself, create solutions, reduce tension, build confidence and bring joy to others.

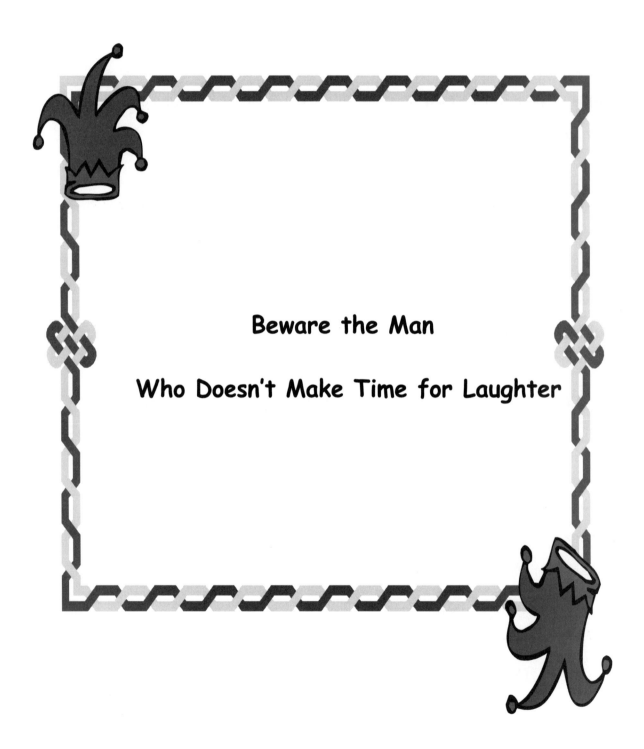

Beware the Man

Who Doesn't Make Time for Laughter

All About or Almost All About Humor

A sense of humor is appreciating and enjoying all the great levity life has to offer. Our culture, our environment, our families and our intellect all trigger humor. Humor is laughing at real life experiences and unexpected daily occurrences. Laughter is universal; we are born with the ability to laugh. After that first cry at birth, you witness babies smiling and laughing for no specific reason. A stand-up comic cannot generate as much happiness and joy as does the pure laughter from babies and toddlers, or anybody else who laughs full heartedly and unconditionally. They laugh because they want to.

Laughter is the best medicine. Laughter expands your vision and gives you a new way of seeing your situation. Laughter focuses us outward instead of inward as tears of sorrow often focus us on self - pity. When you laugh at life and its many dimensions, you are able to acknowledge and accept your own imperfections and move on. **You are accepting reality; you laugh at yourself before others do.** And because you **are accepting reality** through laughter, disadvantages and disabilities become less uncomfortable. Laughter is truly the best weapon against intimidators, bullies and control freaks. You can decide to be happy irrespective of what happens in your life. There's that attitude again!

Talk about last laughs: I'm a professional anything you want me to be. Of course, there is a business dress code for professionals. When I donned the lovable "beanie" hat, my peer professionals wanted to know when the "gag" was over. That lovable "beanie" hat is no gag; it is the best marketing tool I ever used! I make a lot of people smile and want to do business with me. I make their day and they make mine!

What's the payoff? No benefit plan provides a greater value than a daily dose of compassionate humor.   It provides hope, reduces tension, includes all people and creates bonds. Specifically, muscles relax, and stress hormones such as epinephrine, cortisol, dopae, and growth hormone decrease. Your immune system gets a boost with an increase in immunoglobulin A (IgA), a protector against respiratory infections.   After watching 30-60 minutes of a comedy video, salivary and blood levels of IgA are increased. That means you have a stronger defense system against infection. Helper-T - cells and natural killer cells are increased with bouts of laughter and relaxation. Just in case you suffer from arthritis pain, try laughing for at least 10 minutes (you'll have to practice) and you'll wonder where the pain went. There seems to be some magical force that reduces inflammation following robust laughter. Funny thing is you don't need to go to clown school to know how to laugh!   You just have to start saying, "He He, Ha, Ha," smile, and bingo, you're laughing!

And for those of you who need exercise to help prevent or treat cardiac disease, laughter is known as "internal jogging" and is almost as good for lowering resting heart rates as external jogging. The list goes on. Blood

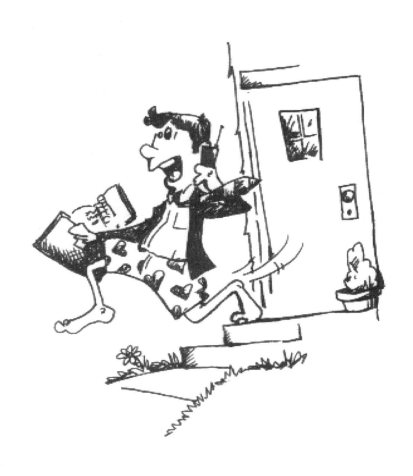

Are You Caught Up In The Hurrying Habit?

pressure decreases, an increase in respiratory exchange occurs with more oxygen coming in and more carbon dioxide going out, and muscles benefit from increased metabolism – all from laughter.

Compassionate humor and laughter is a pension plan with accumulating emotional and cognitive benefits. Not only do you feel good and have fewer episodes of "bad moods," you briefly suspend problems and worries. This is your prescription for anti-anxiety: **play and laugh** before taking a test or presenting a report, and you can then cope with crisis and change. Stress levels are reduced, endorphins are increased and your thinking ability is sharpened. You are now able to take control. You can successfully face problems when you feel good enough to accept the situation with a bit of humor. Always remember to have an attitude of gratitude. It's your choice to react or respond.

Responding by engaging others to laugh helps others feel good about themselves as well. As you laugh with others, you create interpersonal connections and bonds. This results in others liking you alleviating loneliness, boredom and helplessness. Optimism and confidence abound; healing, survival and a passion for living result.

To paraphrase Groucho Marx:

" A Caring Clown Is Like An Aspirin, Only He Works Twice As Fast."

Remember The Riddler

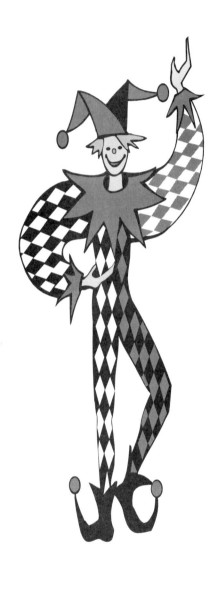

Q. If a dog should loose its tail,
   Where would he go to get another?

A. To WalMart where every thing is
   retailed.

Q. Is it safe to write a letter on an
   empty stomach?

A. It certainly is, but it would be
better to write the letter on paper.

Different strokes for different folks.

Humor comes in different packages. Healthy humor connects and relieves tension. Find one that tickles your funny bone.

Parody: Imperfections are brought to light, such as during a "celebrity roast." Are you old enough to remember "The Dean Martin Celebrity Roast?"

Satire: The expression of exaggerated personal and social flaws. Dave Barry, Erma Bombeck and Art Buchwald are masters of satire.

Slapstick: Physical farce is used to generate laughs. This is aggression-based humor. By watching someone else give and receive physical blows, anger is released by laughing in a cathartic way. The Three Stooges, Lucille Ball and the Marx Brothers demonstrate slapstick comedy perfectly.

Incongruent /Absurdities: Two or more ideas are united which result in a stupid, ludicrous or ridiculous concept. Gary Larson's "The Far Side" is a perfect example. Bill Cosby is a master of pointing out the absurdities of life and Homer Simpson is continuously manifesting life's incongruities!

Dark humor: Based on the fear of death. This kind of humor surfaces during national tragedies or other hard times as a way to cope with gruesome reality. The television show "M*A*S*H" explored these themes with wit and prowess (Also known as "gallows" humor).

Irony: Two concepts or events, when paired come to mean or expose the opposite of the expected outcome. Have you ever ordered apple pie and a diet Coke ™? Did you know Charlie Chaplin once entered a Charlie Chaplin look-a-like contest and won third prize! That is "irony."

Dry humor and puns: Playing with language and/or using words with more than one meaning create verbal humor using personal wit. Simple puns do not have to be very funny to lighten up a stressful situation. You may remember the following old classic moron joke:

"Why did the moron tiptoe past the medicine cabinet? He didn't want to wake up the sleeping pills."

Can Humor Hurt? You Bet It Can!

Putdown humor creates barriers, increases hostility and stress, increases defensiveness, focuses on the negative and increases the potential for disease. **Sarcasm, Caustic or Negative** humor carries a negative attitude and has a negative effect on the beneficiary of the humor. Making fun of someone's mistakes, humiliating someone with humor, name - calling and "mean" practical jokes are just a few ways humor can result in physical and/or psychological harm.

So forget about being a wicked witch - Lighten Up!

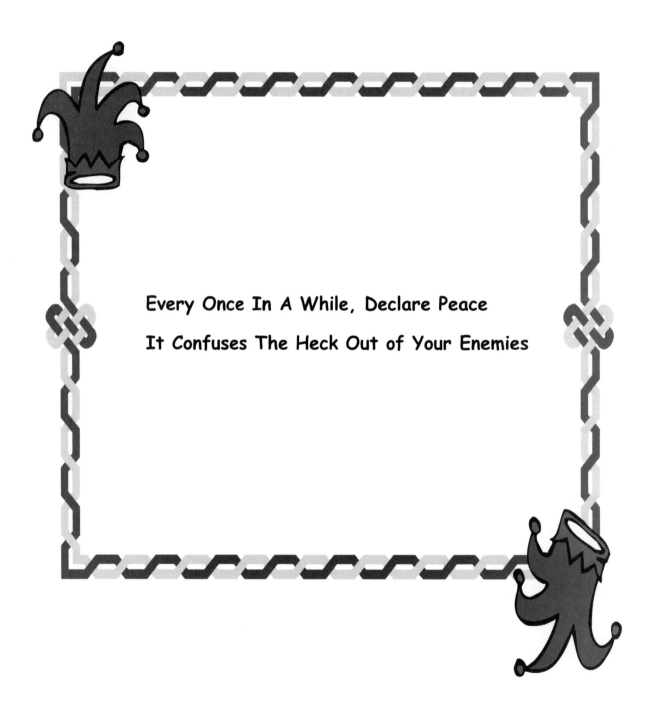

Every Once In A While, Declare Peace

It Confuses The Heck Out of Your Enemies

Try Laughing For The Jest Of It!

To make things even more fun, try laughing in different ways. Who ever thought you could hum laughter with your mouth closed, laugh and clap your

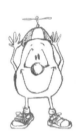

hands in time to your laughs, laugh and dance at the same time, or gradually begin a laugh with a smile, then slowly giggle and continue until the giggles become a full blown hearty laugh? Is this outrageous or what? If you have any desire to get a cheap thrill, begin laughing from deep down in your belly or try one of the aforementioned laughter schemes.

Why Should There Be Humor In The Workplace?

If you're gainfully employed, you are most likely not laughing 9-5, 7-3, 3-11, or 11-7. You could be trapped in the hurry habit, terminal seriousness or professionalism.   However, there are some wickedly good companies out there in the land of capitalism experiencing the benefits of humor and play. Would you believe progressive leaders do exist and even have regard for the human condition as they visualize dollar bills filling their pockets?

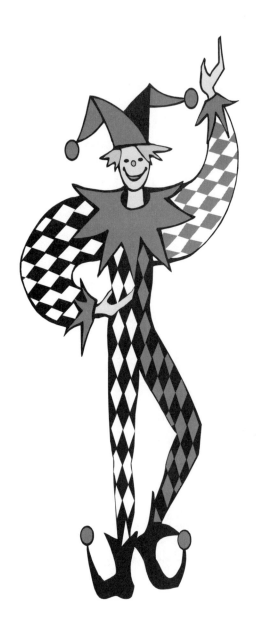

Top Five Reasons "Play" Makes You Successful:

1. You Have Fun Working

2. You Stop Watching the Clock

3. Creates Repeat Business

4. Creates Unbeatable Teams

5. Your Brain Becomes an Honorary Member of Phi Beta Kappa

What are these great leaders discovering about humor in the workplace?

Humor has been added to the list of management strategies to help alleviate job dissatisfaction, stress, absenteeism and increase profits and productivity. The use of play, toys, laughter and creative stimulation linked with employee/employer commitment, coaching and appreciation provide the employee with motivation and increased ability to cope with change. Improving sense of humor on the job prevents burnout and increases self-esteem.

Humor is an effective tool for team building and improving communication skills. Managing with an attitude for fun and humor leads to creative marketing, outstanding customer service, effective conflict management, successful employee motivation and longer retention of talented employees.

CEO's, Managers, and Supervisors what are you waiting for? Take down all of those negative posters and flyers and put up a sign that says:

FUN COMMITTEE NOW FORMING
APPLY WITHIN

"No One Can Make You Inferior Without Your Consent"

-Eleanor Roosevelt

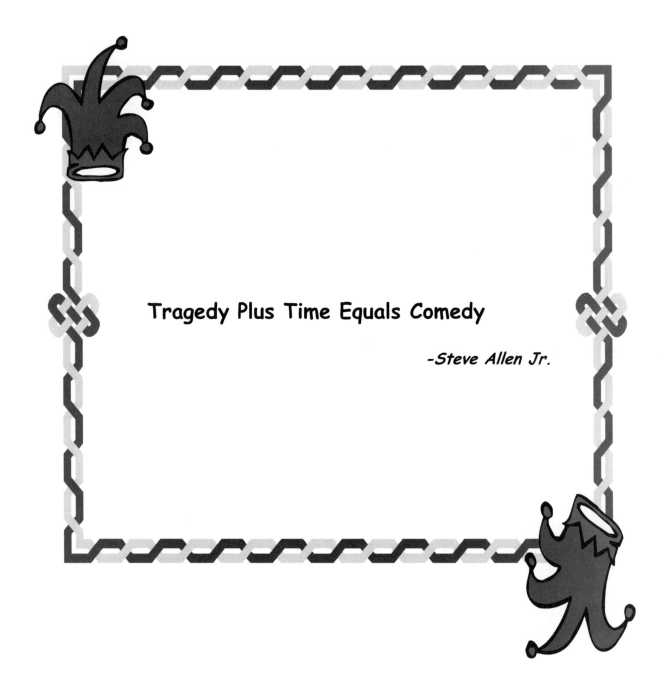

Tragedy Plus Time Equals Comedy

-Steve Allen Jr.

Where's The Humor?

Don't wait for management to initiate humor and play. If you've been putting out fires all day long, have no time to think or take a breath, or stare at the goldfish, you need to escape this cycle. You need to be creative and remain fluid as work - loads increase, deadlines become more frequent and life appears to get tougher. You need to Lighten Up and find that sense of humor. It is not exactly something you call up and order from the local carry - out or pick up on the shopping channel.

Remember, humor is a way of viewing and interacting with the world. It is keeping that inner child alive. With a sense of humor you have a chance to move your life in the direction of health and happiness. You don't have to get caught up in the sea of "toxic niceness." Living with resentment and anger because your friends tell you it isn't polite to laugh loudly and you really like laughing out loud, or saying "yes" when you really want to say "I don't think so" or "absolutely not" is like being sentenced to life in prison.

Break the rules, cut across the grain and challenge the old guard. When it comes to work or societal norms, you are not your work or society's rules. Take yourself lightly. If you're not laughing, you're not doing it right. Humor allows you to stay fluid through it all.

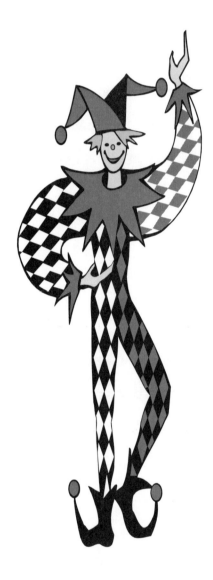

What are 10 Things You Enjoy and Have Fun Doing?

1

2

3

4

5

6

7

8

9

10

How Many of Them Have You Done Recently?

Change your outlook and create your own humor profile.

It's time to find out what really makes you laugh and be as silly as possible. This is where humor becomes serious business again. Answer the following questions and you will find yourself laughing more than 20 times a day.

Let the fun begin!

What makes you laugh at home, at work, on TV, in the movies, in books and cartoons? I hope your list is long!

What are the five funniest movies you ever saw?

What are three of your favorite cartoon strips? Why?

Name two or three people who make you laugh.

What was your favorite story as a child?

When was the last time you read a humorous novel?

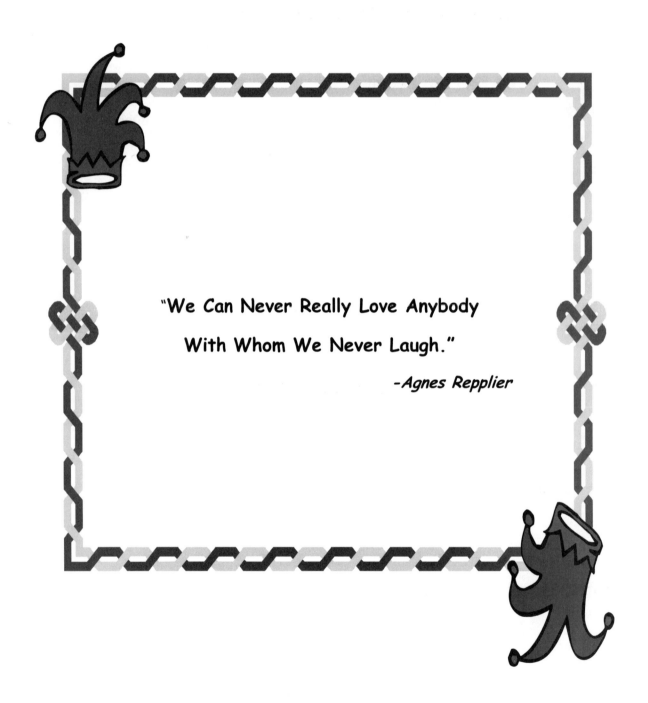

"We Can Never Really Love Anybody

With Whom We Never Laugh."

-Agnes Repplier

When do you laugh the most? Why?

When do you laugh the least? Why?

How long do you hold on to misery before allowing yourself to let loose with humor or laughter?

What stimulates or motivates you to lighten up or let go of your misery?

How many times a day do you laugh?

What did you discover about your use of humor?

If You Are Grouchy, Irritable, or Just Plain Mean, There Will Be A $10 Charge for Putting Up With You!

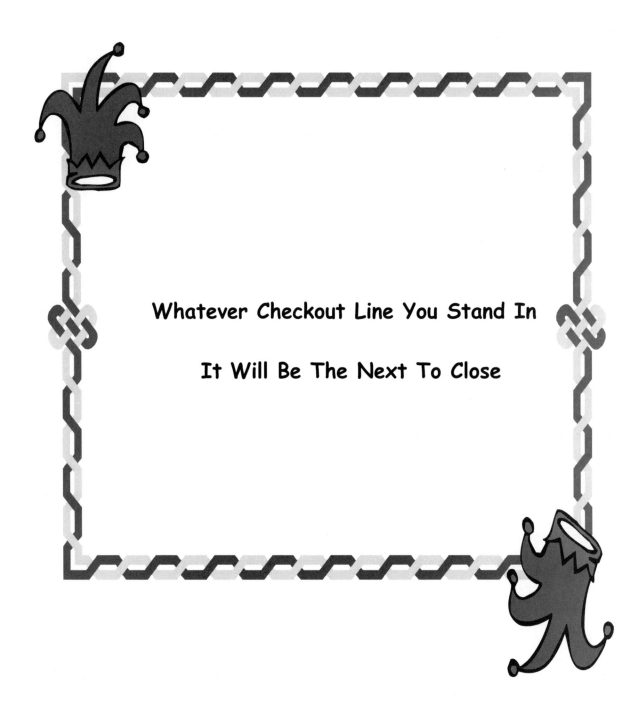

Whatever Checkout Line You Stand In

It Will Be The Next To Close

Where Do You Find Humor?

Humor is everywhere. Everyday situations and surroundings provide an opportunity to play, to be creative and spontaneous. It's all in the eyes of the beholder. First you have to dump the clutter in your head. All that stuff that prevents you from seeing the silly side, being silly or just plain being a fool. Don't forget the fools role is to teach you how not to take yourself too seriously.

 Allow your mind to run wild with ideas when observing every day situations. Watch people and their expressions; it's like watching "Candid Camera." Keep a record of the things that make you laugh or smile. Read it every night before you go to sleep. Soon you won't even know what stress is!

Signs and headlines are always good for a laugh or two. You might see this sign posted at the copy machine in your office:

Tell Me What You Need, And I'll Tell You How To Get Along Without It.

And then again, you might see these meant to be serious but really funny signs in your travels round town.

1. *At the optometrist's office: "If you don't see what you're looking for, you've come to the right place."*

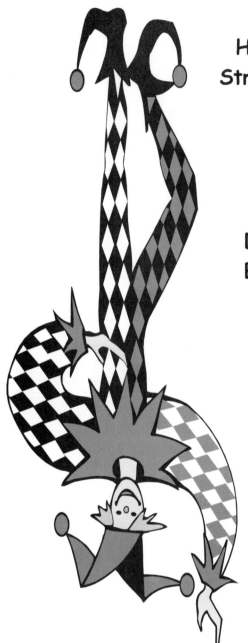

He He, Ha Ha, Ho Ho
Strange Things Are Happening

DON'T WORRY
BE HAPPY

LET A SMILE BE YOUR
        UMBRELLA

HAKUNA MATATA

2. *In the waiting room of the veterinary clinic: "Be back in five minutes. Sit! Stay!"*

3. *On the butcher's window: "Let me meat your needs."*

4. *In a cafeteria: "Shoes are required to eat in this cafeteria. Socks can eat any place they want."*

5. *A bean supper will be held Wednesday evening in the community center, music will follow.*

6. *Weight Watchers™ will meet at 7 PM at St. Johns church. Please use the large double door at the side entrance. How's that for an insult!*

7. Then and Now: Then: A Keg; Now: An EKG

    Then: Acid Rock; Now: Acid Reflux

Look for the absurd, the incongruent and the unusual about your situations. If you have a problem from all that emotional constipation and fear of ridicule, ask yourself what could you change to make the situation funny? Don't aggravate yourself with draining your brain; join the "processing revolution" and let your brain act like a computer. Anything and everything is stimuli. When you need to be creative, to inject a little humor, think creative, imagination and invention. Wild ties, Disney Characters, water balloons, chocolate ice cream, squirt guns, funky hats; anything that makes you think of something else helps you process stimuli into ideas. All you need is an idea to view your situation differently. You can distract yourself from

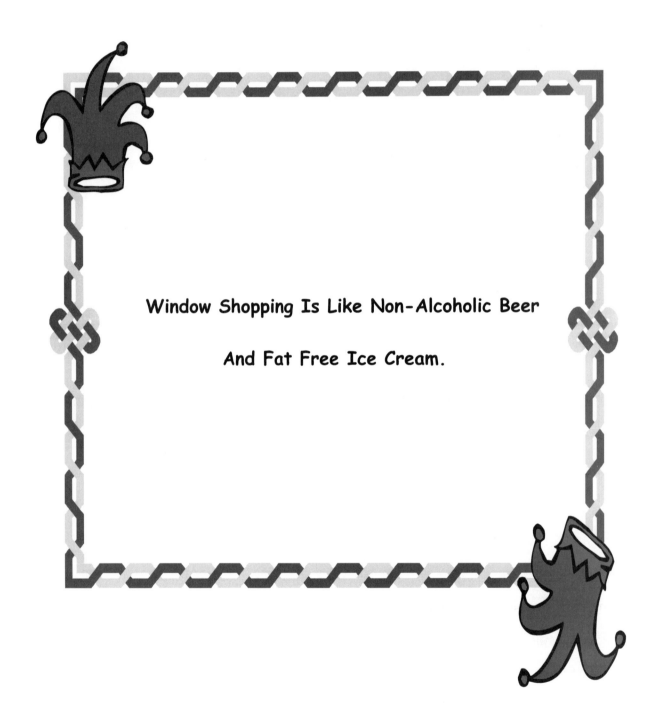

Window Shopping Is Like Non-Alcoholic Beer

And Fat Free Ice Cream.

something you can't control and get to a point where you can do something about it.

If you really want to laugh more, be less, stressed, answer the next two questions in relation to your situation; success is yours. You can change the way you view the world!

1. **What would be the simplest solution?**

2. **What would be the most outrageous solution?**

Patty Wooten author of *Compassionate Laughter, Jest for Your Health* tells a wonderful story about a nurse who was experiencing much frustration because her patient was not producing the desired outcome an enema is known to stimulate. Creativity to wins again. Nurse Nancy grabs a "T" shirt, transforms herself into a cheer leader and calls for the following: "Give me an **S**, Give me an **H**, Give me an **I, and you know the rest of the story.** Yes indeed, laughter was everywhere as was the desired outcome! Just think, if you laughed hard enough everyday, you wouldn't need to think about that fiber product you keep putting in your morning juice.

Want to have fun with an irate customer? Answer a highly technical question in your best Elmer Fudd, Bart Simpson or Donald Duck Voice. The customer will be eating out of your hands!

How To Use Humor All Year Long
Here, There and Everywhere

You've got to begin with yourself. Begin with a smile every day. Even if you fake it, there are benefits. Smiling and laugher make you happier. When you move those facial muscles, messages are sent to the brain changing your emotional state for the better. Some say that smiling cools the brain while frowning heats it up. Just as holding your arms crossed across your chest is a signal not to get too close, a smile is a cue to openness and acceptance. Go ahead and show those teeth. It's a great way to start the day.

If you really want to start the day off right, stand in front of a full- length mirror naked and point that finger at yourself and say "I Love You." Are you laughing yet? When you think of your body do you want to cry or laugh? Let out a great big howl and laugh from deep down in your belly. Try it for a couple of minutes. It will take practice. Your mood sure will change. You won't notice the sad sack you passed in the hall way because you just pictured him standing naked too. Can't help but giggle. You're ready for anything!

Build your personal humor library at home and at work. Remember those questions you answered a few pages back? The ones that asked you about what comedy movies you liked, what comedians you preferred etc.? Now's your chance to go on a shopping spree! Pick up a few videos like *Beverly Hills Cop, or History of the World, Part I,* or a few audiocassettes to keep you laughing while stuck in traffic. You might want to try *All I Know About Animal Behavior I Learned by Erma Bombeck*. You don't need permission to go to the toy store and buy yourself toys you use to love to play with or even new models of Nerf ™ balls, water guns or Koosh™ balls. Don't be a wimp; get a dartboard so you can throw darts at the dartboard representing people who aggravate you. Have a contest with your co-workers to see who scores the highest points. If your kids are really in the talking back phase, visualize them working at the zoo taking care the animals! Most importantly keep small fun reminders around you wherever you are to provide a brief moment of fun, smiles or laughter. If you have memorabilia from a vacation, keep it in your desk drawer or the window - sill in your kitchen. If *Dilbert* tickles your fancy, have a book or two mixed in between your workbooks. Read it when you need to lighten up. Have a collection of small play toys that make you smile like smiley pencil toppers. It's hard not to smile when you are taking notes with a smiley face!

When you need a quick fix to deal with unpleasant situations try visualizing it in the most exaggerated way. Pick any situation and ask yourself what the logical response would be. Then find the opposite of that response, or any of a host of equally wrong answers and you will be humorized, able to gain a new perspective – a new opportunity.

The Magic of A Smile

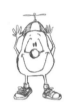

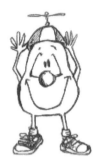

Smiling is infectious
You catch it like the flu
When someone smiled at me today
I started smiling too.

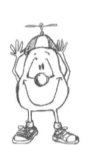

I passed around the corner
And someone saw my grin
When he smiled I realized

I'd passed it on to him

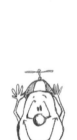

I thought about that smile
Then I realized its worth,
A single smile, just like mine

Could travel round the earth.

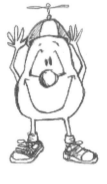

So, if you feel a smile begin,
Don't leave it undetected
Let's start an epidemic quick,
And get the world infected!

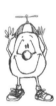

Laughing at yourself creates some of the best humor and opportunities to live life laughing. Accepting your imperfections, joking with others helps others accept themselves as well. Try awarding the biggest bloopers.

Spread the fun to other people. Include everyone in your efforts to lighten – up. Place a jar of different colored jelly - beans on your desk along with a list of which color to take for each kind of stress.

Build your humor library and watch those videos and share those jokes with friends and family. When you laugh with others, you laugh more heartily and enjoy it more.

Get together with co-workers just for fun. Have a funny hat day and award a prize to the most creative.

Keep a collection of foam clown noses in a safe place. When the air gets heavy, grab a nose or two, grab a friend or two and put those noses on. Now walk out in the hall and ask for an autograph. Tension breaks, laughter ensues and you're now having fun at work. You can do this at home too. Put a clown nose on before dinner, during dinner or after dinner. The one thing that's sure to happen everyone will have a good laugh.

Create a fun committee wherever you are. Plan weekly, silly activities like imitating the big cheese contest, dunk the CEO, or bring in a barrel of ice cream scoops for everyone.

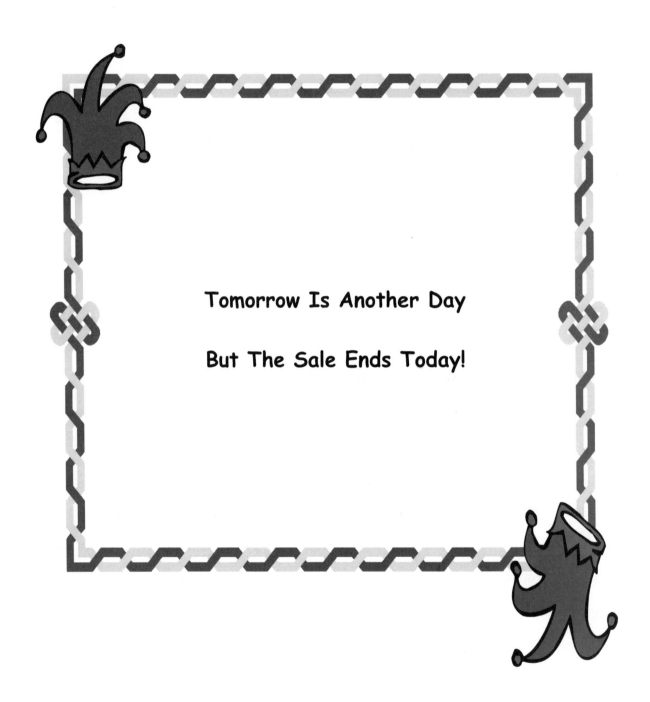

Tomorrow Is Another Day

But The Sale Ends Today!

Have everyone tell what kind of fun they would like in order to make their environment a fun place. See how many ideas can be implemented. Just think you could find your snapshot on the body of National Geographic's featured animals posted on the bulletin board!

Tell jokes before you complain; create an environment that allows you to goof off. Remove barriers to fun.   Build a humor library at work that is shared by everyone. Build a toy box filled with humor magazines, books, videos and toys. Don't delay the fun.

Every night you and your children can write a diary of funny things that you hear each other say. At birthdays or holidays, gift wrap them and see how much fun you have.

Make funny friends. Sounds ridiculous, but when you hang around with funny people, your sense of humor grows, your moods stay elevated and you have a heck of lot more fun daily. The message is don't take life so seriously and never give up.

Start a collection of cartoons, bumper stickers, signs and greeting cards. When you read them out loud, you can't help but crack a smile, make a giggle or just plain laugh.

Keep the child alive! Take an upsetting situation and turn it into an advantage. Christine Clifford, a cancer survivor has used humor to help herself and many others cope with the disease. Her book *Not Now, I'm Having A No Hair Day,* "is a collection of inspirational cartoons for those on chemotherapy, losing hair and weight all at the same time.

When you exaggerate your problem bigger than life to the point of ridiculous, it is easier to find a way to laugh. The problem becomes less threatening. Let me tell you, on the eve of major surgery I am here at the computer finishing this fun book so it can get published on time. I cannot be concerned about the significance of this surgery.

When facing serious or what seem like unconquerable problems, gather friends around and talk about the problems. Make a game. Have everyone randomly call out solutions that come to mind. It doesn't matter if they make sense or not, the sillier, the better. Make them short, unquestioned and absurd. Taste the moment, laugh and the world laughs with you. The problems don't go away, you can handle them more successfully.

If your customers, family or co-workers appear as grizzly bears, visualize them as teddy bears. Imagine their reaction when your response is totally unexpected.

You can never run out of ways to find humor. All you have to do is look for it. Practice and you will have more fun then you could ever dream. Get everyone in a circle, look around wherever you are to see what you can smile about. From now on you will automatically find more things to smile or laugh about.

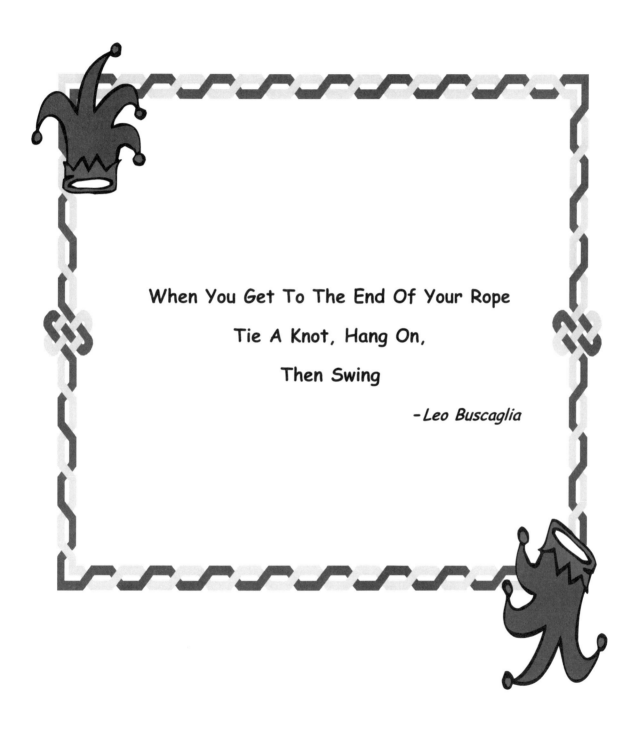

When You Get To The End Of Your Rope

Tie A Knot, Hang On,

Then Swing

-Leo Buscaglia

How the Corporate World Uses Humor

Humor in the workplace is not a dirty word; at least not as much as it use to be. The old guard still believes if you are playing you are not working. You only get paid when you are working.

Our good ole research buddies have done it again. They have demonstrated beyond a shadow of a doubt (and there are many in the corporate world) humor increases profits, decreases absenteeism, stimulates creativity and sharper thinking and above all keeps customers coming back. Humor in the work place has employees coming to work because they want to not just to collect a pay check.

So how are these companies playing?

One of the most famous small businesses incorporating humor and commitment is The Pike Place Fish Market located in the Public Market in Seattle, WA. There a unique environment exists where all of the employees have chosen to choose their attitude to have fun at work. They are there to make the customer's day as well as coach each other in making the best day possible for everyone. You bet; they are throwing fish all over the place. Customers love it. There is an energy surrounding that little stall that cannot be matched anywhere else in the market. Moral is at an all time high and so are sales!

Planning for fun is not just a matter of playing with toys. It is an attitude of choice and a willingness to take risks, do something different to create an experience that has a domino effect. One-person shares that experience with another and before you know it, everyone is letting somebody else be right, and teams are bonding and creating new leadership roles.

There's a bank in Stamford, CT that keeps its employees happy with a frozen T - shirt contest. The goal is to see who can get a frozen T- shirt on the fastest.

Hal Rosenbluth, CEO of Rosenbluth International says, "The only way for us to continuously provide solutions to the needs of an ever – changing business world is to have the kind of environment where spontaneity thrives." Mr. Rosenbluth measures his organization's "happy quotient" by sending out crayons and a blank piece of paper to employees, who draw their current view of the company. He actually compares these drawings every six months to measure any changes in the way people feel about his company.

The famous Eastman Kodak Company makes every day an exciting day. The company hosts such events as Pig Outs, Friday Donut Breakfasts, Casual Day and Halloween Costume Contests. This helps keep creativity and high energy alive.

Newsletters are common vehicles of communication in many companies. One innovative company in Naperville, Illinois asked employees what fun

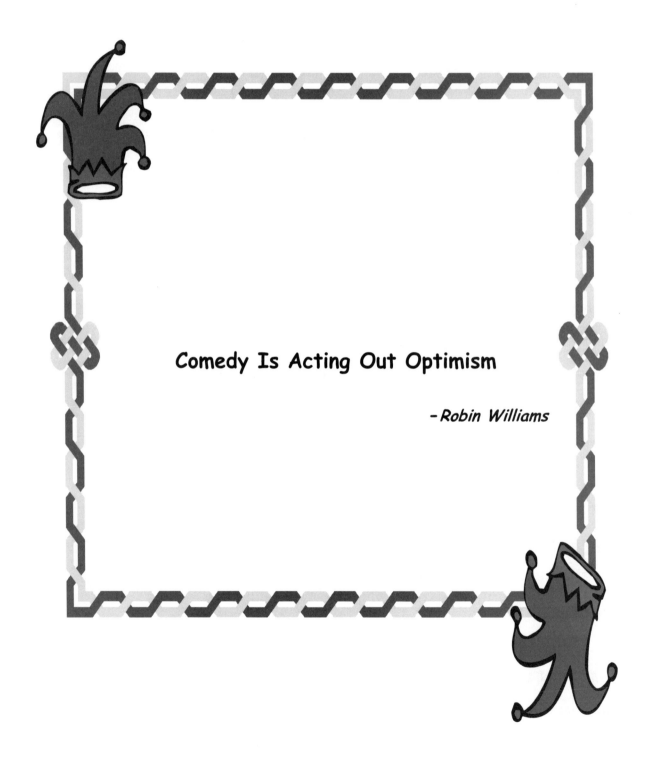

Comedy Is Acting Out Optimism

-Robin Williams

ideas or thoughts they wanted included in the weekly newsletter. They responded with the following ideas:

- ❋ Reviews of local restaurants
- ❋ Movie reviews
- ❋ Crossword puzzles with employee names
- ❋ Jokes
- ❋ Information about what was happening to employees in their personal lives
- ❋ Space for wild and wooly ideas

You would not believe the results. They were measurable!

1. Providing recognition and an opportunity to share and be given credit for ideas raised employee moral.
2. It exemplified the philosophy of taking business seriously and oneself lightly.
3. Employees gained writing and communication skills.
4. It provided an opportunity for employees to connect with one another on a persona level. ("I saw your son made the soccer team.")
5. It gave everyone something to look forward to weekly.
6. The list of movie and restaurant reviews became popular with employees and clients.

Have more effective meetings. Before the meeting starts, distribute a clown nose to all participants and have them put it on. Everyone bursts out in laughter and the goals of the meeting are more efficiently achieved.

What are the most popular toys found in offices today? You got it; clown noses, yoyos, tinker toys, slinky, silly putty, Nerf ™ Balls, Koosh™ balls, Frisbees and Roomarangs.

What do people do with these? They play! They use them to break the tension, to acknowledge mistakes and goof ups, and to reduce the stress of tedious labor. Creativity is increased and employees are happy to come to work.

Dare to Laugh Daily

It's Good For Your Body, Mind, and Soul!

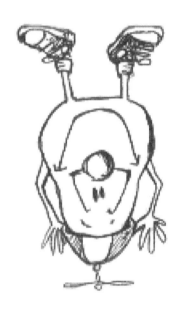

When You Choose Humor,

You Choose To See The World From A Different Perspective

Successful Fun Activities

You Want to Remember

A Recipe For Living

Although the recipe is for a simple thing that we have all tasted before and hope to savor again, it can be elusive at times. The ingredients are to be found in most households and cost next to nothing, but the finished product may require considerable time and effort if you want it to turn out right. I hope that you will make this recipe frequently and will share it with friends and family.

Happiness

Equal parts:

Friends, family, and loved ones

Work you enjoy

Personal growth

The ability to appreciate what you have

Step 1: This is the most important step. Gather around you as many of your loved ones as you possibly can, and do it as often as you possibly can. Make sure that they all know how much you care about them and how much you value your time with them, and you will be rewarded with their love. If friends and family are in short supply, try making new friends, or turn to your favorite animals for companionship. It doesn't matter who you surround yourself with, as long as you love them.

Step 2: Enjoy your work. If you have a job you don't enjoy, try doing something different. This is easier said than done, but life is too precious to spend toiling at something that delivers no satisfaction. If necessary, develop new skills that will enable you to go after the job of your dreams. If changing jobs is not practical and you just can't have a job that you enjoy, then try to enjoy the job that you have.

You will live happier if you do. That's where the humor comes in!

Step 3: Never stop growing. Set time aside to do things that you enjoy. Try doing things you have never done before. Read, learn, study, contemplate, volunteer, lead, follow, experiment, debate, discuss, agree, disagree, challenge, and accept. Those who
cultivate these practices grow better with time, those who do not only grow older.

Step 4: Take time to appreciate your blessings. Take inventory often of the people who love you, of the things that bring you security and happiness, and be thankful in any and every way you can. If your
beliefs include a deity, then direct your thanks to Him or Her. Tell your friends and family how fortunate you are to have them, and remind
yourself at least once a day how wonderful life is.

Step 5: Mix the ingredients in equal portions, or in portions that suit you. Monitor the mixture closely and adjust proportions daily according to your tastes and needs. Serves as many people as will fit in your hopes and your wishes and your heart, so be sure to make enough for everybody. Serve immediately and often.

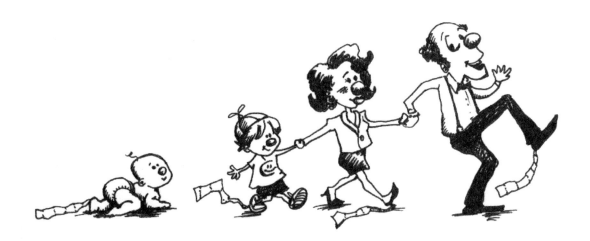

Create A Humor Program

Instead of Coffee Breaks Have a Humor Break

Create a Humor Room A room specifically designed for informal patient or employee support to include lots of laugh sessions and shelves with toys, etc. Allow people to play and talk about anything other than work. This is now a "Stress Free Zone."

It's almost as good as the snack cart but it's a...

Comedy Cart Mobile, humor on a roll, brings mirth aide right next to frightening medical equipment. It contains comedy tapes, toys, smile on a stick, squirt toys, groucho glasses and of course dozens of clown noses and squeaky toys to make you laugh. Comedy Carts are great for senior adult facilities, day care centers, nursing homes, hospitals and assisted living centers. Just in case you live in a big mansion, you've got a mobile entertainment center that brings laughter to everyone.

The Humor Tool Box

Great for birthdays, gag gifts, awards, and get well wishes. The humor tool box is good for everyone. Fill it with your favorite wind-up toys, joke books, cartoons, videos, audio - tapes, puppets, and puzzles. Instructions come with every box to insure stress reduction, increased productivity and innovative ideas for living healthier and happier lives.

Humor Tool Boxes packaged for corporate fun and healing humor can be ordered from: ABC Wellness-Dare To Laugh Workshops (Trieber Associates, Inc.)

Standard gift boxes retail for $19.95 plus $4.95 shipping and handling.

Quantity discounts available

Fax Orders: 410-356-5921

Telephone Orders: 410-998-9585

New Website & E-Mail:
www.humorfusion.com
roz@humorfusion.com

E-Mail Orders:

Postal Orders: Trieber Associates, Inc., P. O. Box 601,

                         Owings Mills, MD 21117-0601

.

Humor Resources

Caring Clown Programs:

Clown Ministry Cooperative; Phoenix Power and Light, Inc. PO Box 820, Oxon

Hill, MD20745

•American Association for Therapeutic Humor

222 S.Meramec, Se. 303, St.Louis, MO 63105, Phone: 314-863-6232

•Carolina Health and Humor Association

Ruth Hamilton: 919-544-2370

5223 Revere Road, Durham, NC 27713

http://www.cahaha.com

Publications

Journal of Nursing Jocularity

PO Box 40416, Mesa, AZ 85274, email: laffinrn@net.com

-Humor and Health Journal

PO Box 16814, Jackson, MS 39236, Phone: 601-957-0075

World Wide Web - Search therapeutic humor

The Laughter Remedy

http://www.laughterremedy.com

Jest for the Health of It

http://www.mother.com/JestHome/

Journal of Nursing Jocularity

http://www.jocularity.com

The Humor Project

http://www.humorproject.com

In Your Face Cards

http://www.inyourface.com

HUMOR$_x$http://www.humorx.com

Add additional websites:

References and Recommended Reading

Bates, Roger. *How To Be Funnier, Happier, Healthier, & More Successful Too!* Cary, North Carolina: Trafton Publishing, 1995

Bedrosian, Maggie. *Life Is More Than Your To-Do List,* Rockville, Maryland: BCI Press, 1995

Goodman, Joel. *Laffirmations.* Deerfield Beach, Florida: Health Communications, 1995

Hall, Doug. *Jump Start Your Brain.* New York: Warner Books, Inc., 1995

Hemsath, D., and Yerkes. L. *301 Ways To Have Fun At Work.* San Francisco: Berrett-Koehler Publisher, 1997

Hilts, Elizabeth. *Getting In Touch With Your Inner Bitch.* Bridgeport, CT: Hysteria Publications, 1994

Hindman, Darwin, A. *Riddles, Riddles, Riddles.* Mineola, New York: Dover Publications, 1997

Jasheway, Leigh Anne. *Don't Get Mad, Get Funny!* Duluth, MN: Pfeifer- Hamilton, 1996

Johnson, Barbara. *Pack Up Your Gloomees in A great Big Box, Then Sit On the Lid and Laugh!* Dallas, Texas: World Publishing, 1994

Kataria, Madan. *Laugh For No Reason*. Mumbai, India: Madhuri International, 1999

Klein, Allen. *The Healing Power of Humor*. New York: Jeremy P. Tarcher/Putnam, 1989

Nelson, Bob. *1001 Ways to Energize Employees*. New York: Workman Publishing, 1996

Vorhaus, John. *From the Comic Tool Box*. New York: Silman – James Pr, 1994

Warren, Roz. *Women's Lip*. Bridgeport, CT: Hysteria Publications, 1998

Weaver, Sherrie. *Shopoholic!,* Glendale Heights, IL: Great Quotations Publishing CO., 1998

Wooten, Patty. *Compassionate Laughter Jest for Your Health*. Salt Lake City, UT: Commune-A-Key Publishing, 1996

Wooten, Patty. *Hart Humor Healing*. Salt Lake City, UT: Publishers Press, 1994

ABOUT THE AUTHOR

Rosalind H. Trieber, MS, CHES, NFL (Naturally Funny Lady)

Rosalind is a health educator turned humorist. She is a humorous and motivational speaker, writer, and a health educator specializing in stress management, humor, and nutrition. Roz has an undergraduate degree in Medical Technology (for which I apologize) and a M.S, CHES, which either stands for a master's of science as a certified health education specialist or might possibly be a master in can't help eating sweets.

Roz is adjunct faculty at Towson University, Towson, Maryland, a contributing writer to Baltimore Health Quest newspaper, co-author of *Life After Schmaltz* (1990) *43 Ways to Keep You and Your Taste Buddies Happy (2000),* and author of manuals used to train health care providers, patients, families, and corporate executives how to use humor to creatively cope with stress, crisis and change.

Roz has created a variety of "Humor Tool Boxes" to help put successful humor strategies in to practice. For information about available products or to schedule Roz to consult or SPEAK to your company, organization, association, or conferences contact:

ABC Wellness - Dare To Laugh
Division of Trieber Associates, Inc.
Workshops for Professional and Personal Success
P.O. Box 601
Owings Mills, Maryland 21117
410-998-9585, fax: 410-356-5921
E-Mail:

New Website & E-Mail:
www.humorfusion.com
roz@humorfusion.com

Order More Books for Family and Friends

Fax Orders: 410-356-5921

Telephone Orders: 410-998-9585

E-Mail Orders: roztrieber@home.

New Website & E-Mail:
www.humorfusion.com
roz@humorfusion.com

Postal Orders: Trieber Associates, Inc., P. O. Box 601, Owings Mills, MD 21117

Please send the following books:

Qty._____ *Live Life Laughing - An Innovative and Imaginative Approach to Living A Healthier, Happier, and Prosperous Life*   @ $14.95

Qty._____ *43 Ways To Keep You and Your Taste Buddies Happy –Outrageous And Hilarious Humor Laced In Between 43 Healthy Delicious Recipes @ $14.95*

Company /Your Name ——————————————————————

Address:_____

City: _____ State:_____ Zip: _____

Telephone:_____ Fax: _____ E-mail: _____

Sales Tax: Please add 5% for items shipped to Maryland addresses.

Shipping & Handling: $4.95 per book

Payment: ☐ Check ☐Credit card: ☐ Discover   ☐ American Express

Total including shipping and sales tax: _____

Card Number: _____ Exp. Date:_____

Name as it appears on card: _____

Signature: _____

Dealer/Gift shop buyer's inquiries invited.   Quantity discounts available.

This book can be used by your organization as a fund-raiser. Please contact Trieber Associates, Inc.